THE HEALING TOUCH

THE HEALING TOUCH

AUGUST RAINES

CONTENTS

Chapter 1: Introduction

For many, illness represents an overwhelming disruption, a formidable adversary. But I've come to perceive it differently: illness, in its myriad forms, is not necessarily unpleasant. At its worst, it's a slight inconvenience. As far as world phenomena go, illness scarcely disturbs my peace of mind. The essence I strive to convey is one of resolution—of healing. However, the price for this resolution is to acknowledge the state of being unhealthy. The most severe form of illness is merely an acute manifestation of unhealthiness.

Personally, my interest lies more in the domain of health than illness. I am drawn to the activities that nurture and enhance health rather than those that seek to cure. The thrill of my contemplation is rooted in the pursuit of feeling good. To an artist, nothing is more captivating than their craft. Similarly, a healthy individual is fervently curious about what the future holds. Every day, I find myself amazed by the capabilities of my body. I want to continue being surprised—to deceive monotony, to flirt with the notion of immortality. The allure of a healthy future is simply irresistible.

This guidebook is as personal as they come. It reflects my unique—and perhaps unconventional—approach to health and healing. My hope is that it speaks to everyone: those who inadvertently create illness, those who endure it, and those who dedicate themselves to healing—doctors, nurses, therapists of all kinds. In my view, every individual in the world falls into one of these three categories. When I speak of illness, I refer to the absence of health. Health, as I understand it, aligns with Kant's profound definition: "the flow of life's energies without impairment and without external interruption."

Arriving at this eclectic approach has taken many years, years filled with deep skepticism about modern orthodox medicine. My journey has been one of questioning established norms and seeking alternative pathways to understanding health. It is a path that has led me to value prevention and wellness above all, to appreciate the body's natural rhythms and capacities.

Health, in my experience, is not just the absence of disease but a vibrant state of being, where life's energies flow unimpeded. It is a dynamic equilibrium, a dance of balance that requires constant attention and care. This book aims to share that journey, to offer insights and practices that can help others find their path to health, to remain curious and engaged with their own well-being, and to embrace the ever-unfolding possibilities of life.

Chapter 2: Understanding Holistic Health

At the heart of holism lies a fundamental principle: **knowledge**. It's crucial not only to understand the mechanisms of systems but also how the different parts of a system interact. This principle underscores the need to look beyond reductionism, which breaks down complex phenomena into simpler parts. While reductionism can provide valuable insights, it often fails to offer a complete understanding of the system as a whole. Many contemporary challenges in medicine and health care stem from this fragmented approach.

General practice, especially in family medicine, is often influenced by narrowly focused specialty knowledge. This tunnel vision can impede the holistic treatment of patients, who need to be viewed and treated as entire systems. For instance, consider a patient undergoing allopathic treatment for heart disease who is also suffering from diabetes. This complex diagnosis might be linked to an unhealthy lifestyle, another domain of allopathic study. Yet, allopathic medicine struggles to connect these disorders and account for existing risks comprehensively.

Holistic health views the body as a network where every organ communicates with the central nervous system, often in response to emotional states. For example, a patient with a severe liver disorder might also suffer from depression, illustrating how physiological conditions can reflect emotional turmoil. This interconnectedness often results in system failures that holistic practitioners aim to address through an integrated approach.

The term **holistic** derives from the Greek word "holos," meaning "whole." Holism views a system as the sum of its parts, existing as a separate, integrated entity. The human body is more than a collection of bones, tissues, and organs; it is infused with vital energies that direct bodily processes. Treating the body holistically means acknowledging this interconnectedness and addressing the individual as a complete entity rather than a series of isolated parts.

In holistic health, practitioners aim to restore balance and harmony within the body. They recognize that physical health cannot be separated from emotional, mental, and spiritual well-being. This approach advocates for the prevention of illness through lifestyle choices, stress management, and natural therapies that support the body's innate healing abilities.

The Philosophy of Holism

Holistic health is rooted in the philosophy of holism, which posits that the whole is greater than the sum of its parts. This philosophical approach can be traced back to ancient systems of medicine, such as Ayurveda and Traditional Chinese Medicine, which emphasize balance and harmony. In these systems, health is seen as a dynamic state of equilibrium, where all aspects of life—diet, environment, emotions—are in balance.

Modern Holistic Practices

Modern holistic practices include a variety of techniques aimed at promoting overall well-being. These can range from nutritional counseling and physical therapies to mindfulness meditation and energy healing. The goal is to support the body's natural healing processes and empower individuals to take an active role in their health.

Holistic practitioners often spend more time with their patients, seeking to understand their life circumstances, stress levels, and emotional health. This comprehensive view helps identify the root causes of illness rather than merely addressing symptoms. By fostering a deep connection with their patients, holistic health practitioners aim to guide them towards a balanced and healthy life.

Chapter 3: The Power of Touch

The human sense of touch is a marvel of biological engineering. At its core are mechanoreceptors, specialized nerve cells that respond to physical pressure or movement. Among these, the most numerous are the free nerve endings and the root hair plexuses, which help us distinguish between different textures—such as recognizing a fabric as rough or smooth—and detect temperature changes, feeling warmth or cold.

When these sensations are experienced, they are processed and transmitted to the thalamus, a central hub in the brain. The thalamus then forwards this information to the somatosensory cortex, where the sensory data is interpreted. However, individuals with sensory symptoms, like numbness or extensive burns, often lack the ability to feel touch with their fine C-tactile afferents. The sense of touch can be classified by the intensity of the stimulus—it can either excite or diminish excitement—and by the role of information transmission from the skin or muscles to the brain, providing insights into the body's position, movement, and temperature.

The Healing Power of Touch

From the first moments after birth to the last days of life, touch has a transformative impact on our physiology, mood, and overall well-being. Studies have shown that touch can alter our physical state and emotional health, underscoring its importance across all stages of life.

The healing power of touch extends to a wide array of healthcare applications. For instance, nurturing touch is essential for premature babies, helping to promote growth and stability. Adolescents struggling with anxiety can find solace and relief through therapeutic touch. Post-surgical recovery can be enhanced by removing adhesions and speeding up recovery times from bruises and minor cuts. General relaxation and stress relief are also significant benefits of therapeutic touch.

The Neuroscience of Touch

Mechanoreceptors in our skin respond to various stimuli and send signals to the brain, where they are processed by the thalamus and the somatosensory cortex. This complex system allows us to experience and interpret different sensations, from the gentlest caress to the firmest pressure. The sensitivity of our skin varies across different parts of the body, influencing our perception of touch.

People suffering from conditions like neuropathy or burns often lose some of their tactile sensitivity, highlighting the crucial role touch plays in our daily lives. For these individuals, the absence of touch can lead to a diminished quality of life, emphasizing the need for therapeutic interventions that can restore or enhance sensory experiences.

Touch in Therapeutic Practices

Holistic health practices often incorporate touch as a fundamental component of therapy. Techniques such as massage therapy, acupuncture, and Reiki aim to harness the power of touch to promote healing and well-being. These practices recognize that touch can facilitate the release of tension, improve circulation, and foster a sense of connection and care.

In massage therapy, different techniques are used to manipulate the muscles and soft tissues, promoting relaxation and pain relief. Acupuncture involves the insertion of fine needles into specific points on the body to stimulate energy flow and alleviate various conditions. Reiki, an energy healing practice, involves the gentle placement of hands on or near the body to balance energy and promote healing.

Conclusion

The power of touch is undeniable and multifaceted. It is a fundamental aspect of human experience, capable of influencing our physical health, emotional state, and overall quality of life. By understanding and harnessing the power of touch, we can unlock new pathways to healing and well-being, ensuring that this vital sense continues to enhance our lives in meaningful ways.

Chapter 4: Techniques for Healing Touch

Our faith in diversity leads us to believe that the knowledge of divinity is not confined to a single text. Instead, it is dispersed through the ancient Vedas, Chinese, Greek, Japanese, and even African wisdom. However, it's important to acknowledge the controversy that sometimes surrounds self-proclaimed healers. Reports of disciplinary actions and legal charges can tarnish the reputation of Healing Touch. This concept, often commercialized and misrepresented as the sole solution, requires discernment. It's crucial not to be swayed by propaganda or become dogmatic followers. Instead, we should seek the best practices and aspire for broad-mindedness.

True healing is often more about the healer's personal and spiritual conduct than the actual technique. Through sustained practice, a healer's sensitivity improves, achieving quicker and more powerful results. This underscores the importance of integrity, empathy, and continuous self-improvement in the practice of Healing Touch.

The Laying-On of Hands

One of the simplest and most natural techniques in Healing Touch is the laying-on of hands. This method has historical roots in various spiritual traditions. Jesus taught this technique to his disciples for healing the sick, as recorded in the Bible. Today, it is known as the Christian Science technique called Treatment, and it is used both for oneself and others.

The laying-on of hands is widely practiced in several faiths and healing systems. Reiki, a Japanese technique, involves channeling energy through the hands to promote healing. The Tibetan technique of Therapeutic Touch focuses on balancing the body's energy fields. Raja Yoga and Pranic Healing also incorporate touch as a means of transferring energy and promoting wellness.

Spiritual and Holistic Techniques

1. **Reiki**: Originating from Japan, Reiki involves the transfer of universal energy through the palms to encourage healing. Practitioners believe that energy can be channeled to stimulate the body's natural healing processes.

2. **Therapeutic Touch**: This technique was developed by nursing professors and is influenced by various cultural practices. It involves the practitioner moving their hands near the patient's body to manipulate the energy field, aiming to restore balance and harmony.

3. **Raja Yoga**: A spiritual practice that incorporates meditation, breath control, and physical postures to balance the mind and body. The touch aspect can be part of guided meditations or energy transfers during advanced practices.

4. **Pranic Healing**: This method involves scanning the body's energy field, cleansing it of negative energy, and replenishing it with positive energy. Practitioners use their hands to direct energy without physical contact.

5. **Yoga Healing and Varmology**: Techniques developed by modern practitioners like Mohan Kharbanda and Ravi Shankar. These methods integrate yoga postures, breathing

techniques, and energy transfer practices to promote holistic healing.

The Role of Tradition and Personal Conduct

While these techniques provide the framework for Healing Touch, the healer's personal and traditional spiritual conduct plays a crucial role. A healer's sensitivity and effectiveness are enhanced through continuous practice, personal growth, and adherence to spiritual principles. This holistic approach fosters trust and reinforces the healing process, benefiting both the healer and the patient.

Healing Touch is a profound practice that spans across cultures and traditions. It integrates ancient wisdom with modern techniques, offering a holistic approach to health and wellness. By embracing diversity and maintaining ethical standards, healers can harness the power of touch to promote healing and enhance the well-being of those they serve.

Chapter 5: Benefits of Holistic Health

In our quest for well-being, we are acutely aware that health is rooted in preventive action. This understanding brings us to the concept of holistic healing, which emphasizes that an individual's health extends beyond the physical. Our well-being also encompasses emotional, intellectual, and spiritual dimensions. It is surprising how what is often considered an illness can profoundly impact one's life, sometimes fatally. Therefore, the concept of healing must evolve to treat not just individual symptoms but the entire system holistically.

This book is a testament to the wealth of indigenous knowledge I have been privileged to grow up with. It draws on various sources, including the direct practices I have experienced, wisdom passed down from my grandfather, and insights from visiting indigenous peoples of Indonesia. The collective wisdom of humanity's diverse cultures is interwoven into the fabric of this book, recognizing that different forms of knowledge can support and enhance each other.

The Dimensions of Holistic Health

1. **Physical Health**: At its core, holistic health acknowledges that physical well-being is fundamental. Preventive measures such as proper nutrition, regular exercise, and adequate sleep are essential to maintaining physical health. These practices help prevent illness and promote a robust, resilient body.

2. **Emotional Health**: Emotional well-being is equally important. Holistic health practices include techniques to manage stress, express emotions healthily, and cultivate positive relationships. Emotional health is integral to overall well-being, influencing how we handle life's challenges and build meaningful connections.

3. **Intellectual Health**: Intellectual stimulation and mental growth are also key components. Engaging in lifelong learning, critical thinking, and creative pursuits keeps the mind sharp and vibrant. Holistic health encourages intellectual curiosity and the pursuit of knowledge.

4. **Spiritual Health**: Spiritual well-being involves finding purpose and meaning in life. This dimension can be nurtured through practices like meditation, prayer, and connecting with nature. Spiritual health fosters inner peace and a sense of belonging to something greater than oneself.

Integrated Approach to Healing

Holistic health approaches healing differently—it is not done in isolation but through a comprehensive treatment of the whole person. This integrated approach considers the interplay between physical, emotional, intellectual, and spiritual aspects of health. By treating the individual as a whole, holistic health aims to restore balance and harmony within the body and mind.

Sources of Wisdom

The knowledge shared in this book comes from a rich tapestry of indigenous practices and traditions. These include not only my personal experiences and those of my grandfather but also the valuable insights from various visiting indigenous peoples of Indonesia. This collective wisdom has been recognized for its ability to support and benefit each other.

The advice and practices outlined in this book are intended to serve as tools for readers to navigate and appreciate the greatness and reality of life. They offer a pathway towards virtue and a balanced, fulfilling existence.

Gratitude and Acknowledgments

I would like to extend my heartfelt gratitude to all the kind individuals whose lives and practices have contributed to this book. My sincerest thanks to those who have been recorded or remain unrecorded in making this book possible. There is an abundance of knowledge that words cannot fully capture. Special thanks to Dr. Joep and Jet van Roosmalen and the dedicated members of the Aymara St. Nicolaas foundation for allowing me to record this invaluable knowledge.

Finally, I recognize that the true guardians of the healing practices shared in this book are the shamans themselves. Their deep care for the well-being of all and their clear understanding that this era is a turning point for our future make their contributions invaluable.

Chapter 6: Creating a Healing Environment

Creating a healing environment is a cornerstone of holistic health. The spaces we inhabit have a profound impact on our physical, emotional, and spiritual well-being. By thoughtfully designing our surroundings, we can enhance our health and promote a sense of calm and balance.

The Importance of a Healing Environment

A healing environment is more than just a physical space; it is a sanctuary that nurtures the body, mind, and spirit. Such an environment helps reduce stress, supports the body's natural healing processes, and fosters a sense of peace and well-being. Whether it is a home, a workplace, or a healthcare facility, creating an environment that promotes healing is essential for overall health.

Key Elements of a Healing Environment

1. **Natural Light and Fresh Air**: Exposure to natural light helps regulate circadian rhythms, improves mood, and boosts vitamin D levels. Ensure that your space has ample natural light and good ventilation. Open windows regularly to allow

fresh air to circulate and consider using air purifiers to maintain clean indoor air.

2. **Colors and Textures**: The colors and textures in your environment can significantly affect your mood and stress levels. Soft, calming colors like blues, greens, and neutrals promote relaxation, while natural textures like wood and stone can create a grounding effect. Use textiles and materials that feel comfortable and soothing to the touch.

3. **Plants and Nature**: Incorporating elements of nature into your space can have a calming and restorative effect. Houseplants improve air quality and add a touch of natural beauty. Consider adding a water feature, such as a small fountain, to introduce the soothing sound of running water.

4. **Sound and Silence**: Create a tranquil auditory environment by minimizing noise pollution and incorporating calming sounds. Soft background music, nature sounds, or white noise can help create a peaceful atmosphere. Ensure there are quiet areas where you can retreat for meditation or relaxation.

5. **Scents and Aromatherapy**: Pleasant scents can enhance mood and promote relaxation. Use essential oils or scented candles with calming aromas like lavender, chamomile, or eucalyptus. Aromatherapy can be a powerful tool in creating a healing environment.

6. **Clutter-Free Spaces**: A cluttered space can contribute to stress and anxiety. Keep your environment organized and free of unnecessary items. Adopt a minimalist approach to decor, focusing on quality over quantity.

7. **Comfortable and Supportive Furniture**: Invest in furniture that is both comfortable and supportive. Ergonomic chairs, supportive mattresses, and cozy seating areas can enhance physical comfort and well-being.

8. **Personalization and Meaning**: Infuse your space with personal touches and items that hold meaning for you. Photographs, artwork, and cherished objects can create a sense of connection and comfort.

Creating Healing Spaces at Home

- **Bedrooms**: Design your bedroom as a sanctuary for rest and rejuvenation. Use calming colors, comfortable bedding, and blackout curtains to create a restful environment. Keep electronic devices to a minimum to promote better sleep.
- **Living Areas**: Arrange furniture to facilitate conversation and connection. Incorporate soft lighting, cozy blankets, and comfortable seating to create an inviting space for relaxation.
- **Bathrooms**: Transform your bathroom into a spa-like retreat with soothing colors, soft towels, and calming scents. Incorporate elements like bath salts, candles, and essential oils to enhance the sense of relaxation.
- **Outdoor Spaces**: If possible, create an outdoor area where you can connect with nature. A garden, patio, or balcony with comfortable seating, plants, and natural elements can provide a peaceful retreat.

Healing Environments in Healthcare Settings

Healthcare facilities can also benefit from incorporating elements of a healing environment. By creating spaces that are welcoming, comfortable, and supportive, healthcare providers can enhance patient outcomes and overall satisfaction. Key considerations include:

- **Patient Rooms**: Design patient rooms with natural light, comfortable furnishings, and personal touches to create a home-like atmosphere.
- **Common Areas**: Create inviting common areas with comfortable seating, natural elements, and soothing colors to foster a sense of community and relaxation.
- **Therapeutic Spaces**: Designate specific areas for therapeutic activities, such as meditation rooms, gardens, or relaxation lounges, to support patient healing and well-being.

Conclusion

Creating a healing environment is a vital aspect of holistic health. By thoughtfully designing our surroundings, we can promote physical, emotional, and spiritual well-being. Whether at home, work, or in healthcare settings, a healing environment fosters a sense of peace, reduces stress, and supports the body's natural healing processes. Embrace the elements of natural light, calming colors, nature, sound, scents, and personalized touches to craft spaces that nourish and heal.

Chapter 7: Nutrition for Holistic Health

The energy of cooked food has a different vibration compared to fresh food. The specific molecules of cooked food vibrate at an altered frequency. To illustrate, the difference between eating raw and cooked food is like the chaotic static of a radio set far between stations versus tuning it to a clear frequency. The sweet taste of raw foods, which aligns with the body's genuine natural cravings, is not nearly as evident as the desire for the opiate effect of sweet sensations, contributing significantly to eating disorders.

To address our blindness to inner needs, we must rekindle our intuitive sense. This sense can guide us through present dangers such as excessive consumption of fats and proteins, and insufficient intake of carbohydrates, vitamin A, vitamin C, iron, calcium, and magnesium.

Understanding Cravings and Nutrition

Our personal relationship with food varies as much as our soul cravings. These cravings often determine what and how much we eat, though they seldom meet the body's true need for nourishment. When the soul is truly nourished, food remains in the stomach longer, saturating cells with life force. Consuming one's "soul food" can increase energy levels by up to 60 percent.

Contrary to popular belief, we do not need as much food as we think. The unfortunate reality is that many of us consume twice the necessary amount of protein and fats, and only half the required carbohydrates. A genuine natural appetite stems from healthy cell nutrition paired with effective digestion. The soul or ego envisions what it considers a meal before desire is kindled. The healthiest meal is one selected by the soul after consulting the body's cellular needs.

The Vibrational Quality of Food

Foods possess different vibrational qualities, which affect their impact on our health. Fresh, raw foods often have higher vibrational energy, promoting better health and vitality. Cooked foods, while easier to digest and often more palatable, may lose some of their vibrational energy during the cooking process. Balancing raw and cooked foods can help maintain a high level of life force energy.

Balanced Nutrition for Holistic Health

Achieving balanced nutrition requires attention to various aspects of diet:

- **Macro and Micronutrients**: Ensure a diet rich in essential nutrients—proteins, fats, carbohydrates, vitamins, and minerals.
- **Whole Foods**: Focus on whole, unprocessed foods that retain their natural nutrients.
- **Variety and Moderation**: Incorporate a wide variety of foods in moderate amounts to avoid overconsumption of any one nutrient.
- **Mindful Eating**: Pay attention to hunger and satiety signals, and eat with mindfulness and gratitude.

Intuitive Eating and Healing

Developing an intuitive approach to eating can reconnect us with our body's true needs. This involves listening to our body's signals and choosing foods that feel nourishing and satisfying on a deeper level. Intuitive eating encourages:

- **Trusting Your Body**: Trust in your body's signals and responses to different foods.
- **Mind-Body Connection**: Strengthening the connection between the mind and body to make healthier food choices.
- **Emotional Balance**: Recognizing and addressing emotional triggers for unhealthy eating patterns.

Conclusion

Nutrition for holistic health goes beyond simply meeting dietary requirements. It involves understanding the vibrational quality of foods, balancing nutrient intake, and developing an intuitive approach to eating. By aligning our diet with the needs of our body and soul, we can achieve greater health, vitality, and well-being.

Chapter 8: Exercise and Movement

The human body is an incredible design, built to defend and celebrate the freedom of movement. Movement is not just a physical necessity but a vital nutrient for our joints, muscles, and overall health. The mission of "Health Liberation" encompasses both the enhancement of our physical shape and the joy of movement. Although these goals might seem contradictory, they are in fact deeply interconnected, built on basic exercises that highlight our unique features and capabilities.

Holistic movement is designed with the intent to improve physical skills, foster awareness of musculoskeletal alignment and posture, and optimize breathing during movements. These practices are health-giving and freedom-enhancing. The ultimate goal is freedom—the freedom to move and to fully embrace the roles we choose in life. We encourage exploration and the discovery of many forms of movement, urging you to travel, investigate, and experiment.

The Essence of Movement

Movement is intricately woven into the human fabric. Our existence depends on constantly shifting, changing postures and movement patterns. Muscle contractions and relaxations lift our bones, flex our spine, enable breathing, heartbeat, eye blinking, and even swallowing around 2,000 times each day. All these are evidence of the energy that flows and changes within us.

Excellence in movement equates to physical skill, yet we are not striving for skill in all things. Skill may have received more credit than it deserves. This doesn't mean we stop moving or that the pursuit of ease and grace in movement diminishes in importance. Rather, for those whose every action already embodies grace, no extra effort is required—movement becomes a natural, unforced expression of life.

Benefits of Exercise and Movement

1. **Physical Health**: Regular exercise promotes cardiovascular health, strengthens muscles, enhances flexibility, and boosts overall physical resilience. Movement is essential for maintaining a healthy body weight, improving bone density, and reducing the risk of chronic diseases.

2. **Mental Health**: Exercise is a powerful tool for mental well-being. Physical activity releases endorphins, which are natural mood lifters. Regular movement can reduce stress, anxiety, and depression, and improve cognitive function and overall mental clarity.

3. **Emotional Health**: Movement helps regulate emotions and fosters a sense of accomplishment and well-being. Engaging in physical activities that bring joy and satisfaction can enhance emotional resilience and stability.

4. **Social Connection**: Many forms of exercise encourage social interaction, whether it's through team sports, group fitness classes, or community events. These connections are vital for a sense of belonging and support.

5. **Spiritual Well-being**: For many, movement practices like yoga, tai chi, and mindful walking can become a form of moving meditation, connecting the body with the mind and spirit. This integration promotes inner peace and a deeper connection with oneself.

Holistic Movement Practices

- **Yoga**: Combines physical postures, breathing exercises, and meditation to enhance flexibility, strength, and mental clarity.
- **Tai Chi**: A martial art that focuses on slow, deliberate movements and deep breathing, promoting balance, relaxation, and energy flow.
- **Pilates**: Emphasizes core strength, flexibility, and mindful movement, improving posture and overall physical health.
- **Dance**: A joyful expression of movement that enhances cardiovascular health, coordination, and emotional expression.
- **Walking and Running**: Simple yet powerful forms of exercise that improve cardiovascular health, strengthen muscles, and provide mental clarity.

Conclusion

Exercise and movement are essential components of holistic health. They nourish the body, mind, and spirit, providing a foundation for overall well-being. By embracing a variety of movement practices, we can enhance our physical skills, foster greater awareness of our bodies, and experience the true freedom of a healthy, active life.

Chapter 9: Stress Management

Stress management is an essential aspect of holistic health, as chronic stress can have severe implications on both physical and mental well-being. The inability to effectively manage stress is often linked to the onset of various diseases, including hypertension, diabetes, cancer, and even heartaches. Acknowledging that stress is an inevitable part of life, it becomes crucial to focus on managing it rather than trying to eliminate it entirely.

The STREZZIMPACY Game

One innovative approach to stress management is the STREZZIMPACY game, a practical tool designed to help individuals identify and enhance their contentment. Unlike theoretical exercises such as lengthy questionnaires, the STREZZIMPACY game involves answering questions related to one's unique knowledge, skills, behaviors, and preferences. Participants repeatedly answer these questions until they are satisfied with their rationale for the events that occurred and their proposed solutions.

The game is structured around five major categories:

1. **Knowledge**: Verbal interaction and understanding.

2. **Skills**: Spiritual, mental, and physical abilities.
3. **Qualities**: Personal traits and characteristics.
4. **Values and Attitudes**: Core beliefs and perspectives.
5. **Beliefs**: Spiritual and personal convictions.

Despite any misused or unused talents, the game encourages participants to believe that their Creator has equipped them with everything needed for life, as inspired by Luke 24:31ff. Goal orientation is emphasized, incorporating practical procedures to tackle challenging situations. The necessary behaviors for overcoming challenges are embedded in the game's design, making it a powerful tool for stress management.

The Concept of PACE

In addition to the STREZZIMPACY game, the concept of PACE (Personalized Approach to Coping and Empowerment) offers a human-focused approach to managing stress. This concept addresses the unique needs of individuals, helping them navigate stress effectively. The latest version of the STREZZIMPACY game (Version 9.11) integrates these principles, offering a more comprehensive tool for stress management.

Principles of Stress Management

1. **Acknowledgement of Stress**: Accept that stress is a natural part of life. It's essential to understand that experiencing stress is not the issue; failing to manage it effectively is.
2. **Practical Strategies**: Use practical tools like the STREZZIMPACY game to identify stressors and develop personalized coping mechanisms.
3. **Goal Orientation**: Set clear, achievable goals to navigate stressful situations. Having a sense of purpose and direction can alleviate feelings of overwhelm.

4. **Mindfulness and Relaxation**: Incorporate mindfulness practices and relaxation techniques to reduce stress and promote mental clarity.
5. **Physical Activity**: Engage in regular physical activity to release built-up tension and improve overall well-being.
6. **Support Systems**: Build strong support networks of friends, family, and professionals to provide emotional and practical support during stressful times.

Stress Management in Different Contexts

The principles of individual stress management are applicable in various contexts, including both secular and religious perspectives. Dr. Hartl's wealth management seminar, for example, incorporates these principles from both a secular and Christian viewpoint, demonstrating their versatility and effectiveness across different areas of life.

Conclusion

Stress management is a vital component of holistic health, requiring practical tools and strategies to navigate life's inevitable stressors. The STREZZIMPACY game and the concept of PACE provide innovative approaches to identifying and managing stress, promoting overall well-being and resilience. By acknowledging stress and utilizing effective management techniques, individuals can enhance their contentment and navigate the challenges of life with greater ease.

Chapter 10: Emotional Well-being

Emotions are the vibrant hues that color our lives, defining and helping to form our personalities. They generate energies that can heal and provide us with transcendental knowledge. Our minds and bodies hold the keys to unlocking our potential abilities, enabling individuals to grow and mature beyond the limitations of the physical body and the emotional mind.

The Healing Power of Emotions

Emotions are meant to be felt and expressed. When properly acknowledged and processed, they can lead to profound healing. Responsible, informed, and caring healers can guide us through the exploration of our emotions, helping to uncover the sources of our anxieties, fears, and anger. By understanding and integrating these feelings, individuals can embark on a positive learning process that leads to personal growth and the transcendental path.

The Body-Mind Connection

The physical body often mirrors our internal state. For instance, individuals who are overworked and unable to cope with life's demands may hide their worries, fears, and anger beneath a facade of false cheerfulness. This can mask the true extent of their distress until the body sends out alarm signals in the form of pain or incapacity, forcing them to pause and reflect.

Some people may struggle to reveal their true nature through conversation or body language, stifling or suppressing their emotions. This suppression can lead to misunderstandings and negatively impact relationships, both professionally and personally. Recognizing and expressing emotions authentically is vital for maintaining healthy and meaningful connections.

Steps to Enhance Emotional Well-being

1. **Self-Awareness**: Develop an awareness of your emotions and how they impact your thoughts and behaviors. This involves regularly checking in with yourself and acknowledging your feelings without judgment.

2. **Expression and Communication**: Find healthy ways to express your emotions, whether through talking to a trusted friend, journaling, or engaging in creative activities. Clear communication helps in building stronger relationships and understanding.

3. **Mindfulness and Meditation**: Practice mindfulness and meditation to stay present and manage stress. These techniques can help calm the mind and enhance emotional regulation.

4. **Physical Activity**: Engage in regular physical activity to release built-up tension and improve mood. Exercise has been shown to reduce symptoms of anxiety and depression.

5. **Healthy Relationships**: Foster healthy relationships that provide support, understanding, and mutual respect. Surrounding yourself with positive influences can enhance emotional well-being.

6. **Professional Support**: Seek guidance from mental health professionals when needed. Therapists and counselors can provide tools and strategies to navigate complex emotions and life challenges.

Embracing Emotional Intelligence

Emotional intelligence involves recognizing, understanding, and managing our own emotions, as well as empathizing with others. It is a key component of emotional well-being and includes:

- **Self-Regulation**: The ability to manage and respond to emotions in a healthy way.
- **Motivation**: Using emotional insight to drive personal and professional goals.
- **Empathy**: Understanding and sharing the feelings of others, which enhances relationships.
- **Social Skills**: Building and maintaining healthy interactions and relationships.

Conclusion

Emotional well-being is a vital aspect of holistic health, encompassing the full range of human emotions and their impact on our lives. By developing emotional intelligence and adopting healthy practices for expressing and managing emotions, we can achieve greater overall well-being. Embracing our emotions and understanding their role in our lives allows us to grow, heal, and connect more deeply with ourselves and others.

Chapter 11: Spiritual Connection

Spiritual connection is not about reaching out to external entities, but about connecting with the pure and good part within ourselves. This stage, though challenging, is profoundly effective. We often refer to a higher power, a being we call God, who resides in heaven. This connection aligns us with our true selves, empowering us and, by the gravitational force of spiritual laws, making us become what we deeply believe in.

When our intentions are continuous and not ceased by death, we can master incredible feats like flying, transportation, and materialization. Conversely, negative intentions can materialize unwanted events and outcomes, aligning with the infernal domain. The earth reflects our subconscious beliefs, evidenced by the aggressive responses of an unhappy nature.

The Ultimate Stage of Holistic Health

Connecting with our true selves and the absolute represents the ultimate stage of holistic health. This stage is characterized by intense self-connection, self-realization, and integrating all the aspects of holistic health described earlier. It involves working through positive affirmations and intentions towards the absolute, where all intentions manifest as realities. In this stage, we tap into the miraculous power of the mind, experiencing empowerment and belief in the unseen (metaphysical).

Transforming Intentions to Divine Models

In this context, our intentions are transformed into divine component models, which are equivalent to our spirits. Everything on Earth grows and evolves according to these set divine models inherent in the atoms that compose things. These models transform feelings of stress, anxiety, and hopelessness into positive, renewing energy and a sense of self-responsibility.

Steps to Foster Spiritual Connection

1. **Inner Reflection**: Regularly take time for introspection and self-reflection to understand your inner self and spiritual beliefs.

2. **Meditation and Prayer**: Engage in meditation and prayer to connect with the divine and cultivate a sense of inner peace and guidance.

3. **Positive Affirmations**: Use positive affirmations to reinforce your beliefs and intentions, aligning them with the greater good.

4. **Mindfulness Practices**: Practice mindfulness to stay present and connected with your spiritual self, enhancing awareness and clarity.

5. **Community and Support**: Join spiritual communities or groups that resonate with your beliefs to share experiences and gain support on your spiritual journey.

6. **Nature Connection**: Spend time in nature to feel a deeper connection with the universe and the natural world around you.

The Power of Belief and Manifestation

Belief plays a crucial role in spiritual connection. Our subconscious mind is a powerful tool that can manifest our deepest beliefs and intentions into reality. By aligning our beliefs with positive and empowering thoughts, we can create a life filled with purpose, joy, and fulfillment.

Conclusion

Spiritual connection is the pinnacle of holistic health, integrating physical, emotional, mental, and spiritual aspects into a harmonious whole. By connecting with our true selves and the divine, we unlock the power to transform our lives and manifest our highest intentions. This journey towards spiritual connection fosters a sense of peace, empowerment, and an unwavering belief in the unseen, guiding us towards a fulfilling and enlightened existence.

Chapter 12: Integrating Traditional and Alternativ

The hallmark of alternative medicine is the integration of philosophy and traditional medical practices, rooted in philosophical and sociological principles. This approach takes special care and attention to the "wholistic" individual. The term "wholistic" derives from the root word "whole," meaning the entire person. Wholistic health practitioners aim not only to address the symptoms reported by the patient but also to examine their lifestyles, emotions, spiritual beliefs, and personal remarks made during the interview process.

The Wholistic Approach

A wholistic approach is characterized by:

1. **Comprehensive Assessment**: Looking beyond symptoms to understand the patient's overall well-being.
2. **Lifestyles and Emotions**: Considering how daily habits and emotional states influence health.
3. **Spiritual Beliefs**: Acknowledging the role of spirituality in healing and well-being.

4. **Personal Interaction**: Valuing the patient's voice and personal insights during consultations.

Integrating Traditional and Alternative Medicine

The integration of alternative medicine with traditional allopathic approaches is an emerging practice. This integrated approach considers the growing interest in alternative medicinals, prompting a desire to learn about their uses, cost-effectiveness, and benefits.

- **Alternative Medicine**: Focuses on natural remedies and holistic practices, including herbal medicine, acupuncture, and mind-body techniques.
- **Traditional Medicine**: Emphasizes evidence-based treatments and interventions, typically involving pharmaceuticals and surgical procedures.

Collaborative Care

Patients may receive treatment from a single provider or a collection of providers using an integrated approach. This collaborative care model combines the strengths of both traditional and alternative medicine to offer personalized and comprehensive treatment plans.

The Historical Perspective

Since the beginning of time, people have been healing themselves and others by utilizing the earth's gifts and their unique capabilities and energies. The earth's layers—sand, rocks, soil, moss, and plants—mirror the complexity and beauty of the human soul and physical being. Each layer of the earth contributes to the overall landscape, just as various tools and practices contribute to our health.

The Layers of Healing

Within each individual's existence, there are many tools that can shape or change lives. Just as one tool alone is never the answer to every problem, multiple approaches often provide the most comprehensive solution. The answer to health challenges is often buried deep within the layers of ourselves, requiring a multifaceted approach to uncover and address.

Benefits of an Integrated Approach

1. **Comprehensive Care**: By combining traditional and alternative medicine, patients receive a broader spectrum of care that addresses both symptoms and root causes.
2. **Personalized Treatment**: Integration allows for treatments tailored to the individual's unique needs and circumstances.
3. **Enhanced Well-being**: Patients often experience improved overall well-being when their physical, emotional, and spiritual needs are all addressed.
4. **Increased Patient Satisfaction**: Many patients appreciate having access to a wider range of treatment options and feel more involved in their care.

Conclusion

Integrating traditional and alternative medicine represents a holistic and inclusive approach to health care. It recognizes the value of both systems and strives to provide comprehensive care that addresses the whole person. By embracing this integrative model, we can unlock new pathways to health and healing, honoring the complexity of human existence and the richness of our diverse medical traditions.

Chapter 13: Holistic Health for Children

When it comes to children or teenagers who do not exhibit any actual symptoms but seem "different," absent-minded, or unable to keep up with their peers, it's crucial to address these signs with care and understanding. Rather than jumping to conclusions or searching for a disease that needs a remedy, our focus should be on helping them reintegrate into a fulfilling life, preventing feelings of bitterness or superfluity.

The Role of Health Inspectors and Educators

Health inspectors, in collaboration with participants in neohumanistic education, are well-equipped to oversee the healthy development of children. Their goal is to support growth without forcing or accelerating it unnaturally. By adopting a holistic perspective, they ensure that children are nurtured in all aspects of their development.

Developing Strength in Body and Personality

The objective in treating children is to help them develop both physical strength and strong personalities. Traditional, rigid methods are often out of place in this context. The very concept of childhood ill health can be misunderstood, especially when adult medical criteria are inappropriately applied to children. Standardized, industrialized medicine often focuses narrowly on organic lesions and physical symptoms, missing the broader picture.

A New Perspective on Childhood Illness

A holistic approach aims to view children "in a new light," interpreting episodes of illness or malaise not as indicators of something fundamentally wrong, but as opportunities to remove obstacles that hinder growth. Whether dealing with general unwellness, periods of suffering, or illnesses that impede development, the therapeutic goal is to clear these obstacles and support the child's natural progression.

The Importance of a Supportive Environment

Creating a supportive environment is key to holistic health for children. This involves ensuring that children feel understood and valued, and providing them with the resources they need to thrive. Emotional and psychological support is as important as physical health care. Encouraging open communication, fostering a sense of security, and promoting healthy relationships all contribute to a child's well-being.

Practical Steps to Support Holistic Health

1. **Observation and Understanding**: Pay close attention to children's behavior and emotional states. Look for underlying causes of distress rather than simply addressing symptoms.

2. **Non-judgmental Support**: Provide a safe space for children to express their feelings and thoughts without fear of judgment or dismissal.

3. **Balanced Approach**: Integrate physical, emotional, and mental health care. Encourage activities that promote physical health, such as exercise and nutritious eating, alongside those that support emotional and mental well-being.

4. **Collaborative Care**: Work with a team of educators, health professionals, and caregivers to create a comprehensive support system for the child.
5. **Personalized Care**: Recognize that each child is unique and tailor care to meet their individual needs and circumstances.

Conclusion

Holistic health for children requires a comprehensive, empathetic approach that addresses the full spectrum of their developmental needs. By viewing each child as a whole person and focusing on removing obstacles to their growth, we can help them achieve their full potential. This approach fosters resilience, strength, and a sense of well-being that will serve them throughout their lives.

Chapter 14: Holistic Health for Seniors

Harmony in the context of holistic health for seniors involves considering the whole community of beings and the abiotic environment. Traditional orthodox medicine focuses on combating disease, infection, and abnormality but often neglects the pursuit of overall health. A more effective approach involves making simple adjustments in our life processes, moving towards a "back-to-nature" philosophy. In this model, healthcare is necessary mainly for addressing injuries, while the broader concept of health care emphasizes a deeper commitment to health rather than disease.

The Holistic Approach

Holistic health practices differ significantly from orthodox healthcare, which is an incomplete system influenced by political, social, and historical processes. Orthodox medicine tends to be disease-centric, focusing primarily on treating specific ailments rather than the wholeness of beings. In contrast, holistic health for seniors aims to:

1. **Promote Overall Well-being**: Emphasize the importance of a balanced life that integrates physical, emotional, mental, and spiritual health.
2. **Prevent Disease**: Focus on preventive measures and healthy lifestyle choices to maintain well-being and reduce the risk of illness.
3. **Natural Healing**: Utilize natural and non-invasive methods to support the body's innate healing abilities.

Integrating with Nature

A fundamental aspect of holistic health is aligning our lifestyles with nature. This approach includes:

- **Diet**: Encouraging a diet rich in natural, whole foods that are minimally processed.
- **Physical Activity**: Promoting regular physical activity that is in harmony with the body's natural rhythms, such as walking, yoga, and tai chi.
- **Mental Health**: Incorporating practices like meditation and mindfulness to maintain mental clarity and reduce stress.
- **Environmental Interaction**: Spending time outdoors to connect with nature and benefit from the healing effects of natural environments.

Addressing Senior-Specific Needs

Seniors have unique health needs that must be addressed holistically:

- **Mobility and Strength**: Focus on maintaining and improving mobility and strength through gentle exercises and physical therapy.

- **Mental Sharpness**: Engage in activities that stimulate cognitive function, such as puzzles, reading, and social interactions.
- **Emotional Support**: Provide emotional support through community involvement, therapy, and strong social networks.
- **Chronic Conditions**: Manage chronic conditions with a combination of traditional treatments and complementary therapies, like acupuncture and herbal medicine.

The Role of Community

Holistic health for seniors also emphasizes the role of community. A supportive community can provide:

- **Social Connections**: Foster social connections to reduce loneliness and enhance emotional well-being.
- **Shared Resources**: Access to shared resources, such as community gardens, wellness programs, and group activities.
- **Intergenerational Relationships**: Encourage intergenerational interactions to share knowledge and experiences, benefiting both seniors and younger generations.

Conclusion

Holistic health for seniors is about embracing a comprehensive and compassionate approach that addresses the whole person. By integrating natural living principles, focusing on prevention, and fostering strong community ties, we can create an environment where seniors thrive in health and harmony with the world around them. This holistic perspective not only enhances individual well-being but also contributes to the balance and health of the broader community and ecosystem.

Chapter 15: Holistic Health for Women

The personal lives of many women often reveal a diminishing life force. Teenage years can deplete the emotional strength of girls who prematurely transition from dependent children to pseudo-independent college students. This premature shift often leads to a superficial lifestyle that takes hold well before their 20s. If the educational phase doesn't take its toll, the tensions of new marriages and childbearing responsibilities add further strain.

The Myth of 'Natural' Childbirth

The concept of 'natural' childbirth is often portrayed as the ideal, particularly for the working class and lower middle class, who may see it as their only viable option. However, this notion can be misleading and fails to address the physical and emotional well-being of women. In the race of life, both the physical and emotional health of women are at stake, as is the sanctity of the reproductive process. Femininity, the most vital natural force in the universe, is seldom nurtured.

Health and Aging

As women approach the age of forty, they often become "health statues," appearing older and frailer than their years. They frequently experience health issues with unclear diagnoses, leading to greater care of appearance without improvement in well-being. This cycle ultimately undermines their self-confidence.

The Emotional Body

A woman's life and health revolve around the strength of her emotional body. Yet, few recognize or nurture the subtle emotional needs of women. Societal and familial structures have conditioned women to excel academically, support the family, and later become submissive wives and good mothers. This societal pressure forces women to suppress their femininity, both in public and at home, where the husband often assumes a paternalistic role.

Recognizing Health Issues

Women who suddenly develop health problems often don't know the cause, nor does anyone else. Family physicians can sometimes be paternalistic or curt, not taking women's complaints seriously because they are not perceived as life-threatening. This lack of understanding can lead to unaddressed health issues and emotional distress.

Steps to Enhance Holistic Health for Women

1. **Recognizing Emotional Needs**: Acknowledge and nurture the emotional needs of women. Emotional well-being is critical to overall health and should not be overlooked.

2. **Supportive Healthcare**: Foster a supportive healthcare environment where women feel heard and their concerns are taken seriously. Empathetic and comprehensive healthcare practices can make a significant difference.

3. **Work-Life Balance**: Encourage a balance between professional responsibilities and personal life. Support systems both at work and at home are crucial.

4. **Empowerment and Self-care**: Promote self-care practices that empower women to take charge of their health and well-being. This includes physical activities, healthy eating, and mental health care.

5. **Community and Connection**: Build communities where women can share their experiences and support each other. Strong social connections contribute to emotional and mental well-being.

Conclusion

Holistic health for women encompasses a comprehensive approach that addresses physical, emotional, and spiritual well-being. By recognizing and nurturing the unique needs of women, we can help them achieve a balanced and fulfilling life. Empowering women to embrace their femininity and providing supportive healthcare environments are crucial steps towards this goal.

Chapter 16: Holistic Health for Men

A holistic approach to men's health includes family planning skills and modern practices that lead towards healthy behaviors. It emphasizes the need to escape from the "cake-icing syndrome" in managing health care services, among other activities. The evolutionary aspects of sexual attraction and behavior are particularly interesting. Sexual activities often open the door to various life pleasures through their association with natural, widespread, and pleasurable activities, linked to fertilization in the animal kingdom. Achieving a comfortable sexual life is crucial for the continued good health of mankind.

Unique Health Needs of Men

Men and women have distinct health needs and face different problems, many of which are behaviorally related. Men, for instance, are often naturally driven to more total activity and movement compared to women, who typically exhibit more placid behavior in daily life-supporting activities. This difference in lifestyle can affect various aspects of health.

Physical Activity and Movement

Men's higher levels of physical activity and movement are beneficial for maintaining cardiovascular health, muscle strength, and overall fitness. Encouraging regular exercise and an active lifestyle can help prevent chronic conditions such as heart disease and diabetes. However, it's also important to balance physical activity with adequate rest and recovery to avoid overexertion and injury.

Sexual Health and Relationships

Maintaining a healthy and fulfilling sexual life is vital for men's well-being. As men age, sexual interests can remain strong, but there may be challenges such as impotence and decreased libido. Providing an enriched social and rural environment can support the continuance of a healthy sex drive. Educated practices promoting balanced male-female relationships are essential for restoring harmony in partnerships and ensuring mutual satisfaction.

Emotional and Mental Health

Emotional and mental health is equally important for men. Society often places pressure on men to be strong and stoic, which can lead to suppressed emotions and mental health issues. Encouraging open discussions about feelings, stress management techniques, and seeking professional help when needed can improve emotional well-being.

Family Planning and Reproductive Health

Family planning is a crucial aspect of holistic health for men. Educating men about contraception, sexual health, and reproductive responsibilities helps in promoting responsible behavior and preventing unintended pregnancies. It also fosters healthy partnerships where both partners are involved in family planning decisions.

Social and Environmental Factors

Special attention must be directed towards creating a supportive environment for men. This includes:

- **Healthy Relationships**: Building strong, positive relationships with family, friends, and partners.
- **Community Engagement**: Encouraging participation in community activities and social networks to combat isolation.
- **Work-Life Balance**: Promoting a balance between work and personal life to reduce stress and improve quality of life.
- **Rural and Urban Health**: Addressing the unique health needs of men in both rural and urban settings, providing access to necessary resources and support.

Conclusion

Holistic health for men involves a comprehensive approach that considers physical, emotional, mental, and social well-being. By addressing unique health needs, promoting healthy behaviors, and fostering supportive environments, we can enhance the overall health and quality of life for men. This holistic perspective not only benefits individual men but also contributes to the well-being of families and communities.

Chapter 17: Holistic Health for Mental Health

Worry is a dangerous factor in mental hygiene. In the relentless pursuit of material wealth, many are betrayed by ambition, never finding peace of mind or lightness of step. Those who achieve their material goals often do so at the expense of their mental well-being, sacrificing mental balance, moral integrity, and the simplicity of life.

The Impact of Lifestyle on Mental Health

Irregularities in life, contrary to natural methods, are primary causes of worry. Late nights, loss of sleep, and discomfort in healthy sleep build deep-seated fatigue without relaxation. These habits contribute to chronic anxiety and mental strain. Rising early, engaging in physical activity such as gym exercises or morning walks in fresh air, and maintaining a balanced lifestyle are essential for mental well-being.

Even moderate exercise is sufficient; intense, rapid exercises beyond a certain efficiency are unnecessary and can be detrimental. Health is a necessity, and the rule is to indulge in it without sacrificing well-being. Overindulgence in physical activities or work can lead to lifelong consequences.

The Influence of Diet on Mental Health

The state of the mind is significantly influenced by the foods we consume. Junk food, excessive alcohol, coffee, and tea can lead to mental disturbances. Even the excessive consumption of natural, innocent foods can create similar issues due to overindulgence. Drinking too much water or any type of beverage at all times can result in a lack of sense and strength in the morning. In contrast, drinking water only when thirsty and stopping when the thirst is quenched prevents harm.

Balanced Diet and Mental Health

A balanced approach to diet is essential for mental and spiritual health. Attention to moderation and the quality of food can prevent it from becoming a cause of intoxication and instead provide mental and spiritual benefits. Consuming a diet rich in whole, unprocessed foods, maintaining hydration, and avoiding stimulants and excesses can support mental clarity and emotional stability.

Practical Steps for Enhancing Mental Health

1. **Establish a Routine**: Create a consistent daily routine that includes regular sleep patterns, balanced meals, and physical activity.
2. **Prioritize Sleep**: Ensure adequate, quality sleep to prevent mental fatigue and support cognitive function.
3. **Moderate Exercise**: Engage in regular, moderate exercise to boost mood and reduce anxiety.
4. **Balanced Diet**: Focus on a balanced diet that avoids excessive stimulants and alcohol, and includes nutritious, whole foods.
5. **Mindfulness and Relaxation**: Incorporate mindfulness practices, relaxation techniques, and stress management strategies into daily life.

6. **Seek Support**: Don't hesitate to seek support from mental health professionals when needed. Professional guidance can help manage stress and mental health conditions effectively.

Conclusion

Holistic health for mental well-being involves addressing the interconnected aspects of lifestyle, diet, and routine. By adopting healthy habits, managing stress, and seeking balance, we can support and enhance our mental health. Recognizing the importance of mental hygiene and making conscious choices to maintain it is crucial for overall well-being.

Chapter 18: Holistic Health for Chronic Illness

Holistic thinking is integral to functional medicine, which personalizes treatment by supporting the body's unique functions, including digestion, absorption, microbiome balance, detoxification, biotransformation, and repair and maintenance. Practitioners utilize a variety of techniques such as diet and nutrition counseling, digestive enzymes, prebiotics, probiotics, and even ultraviolet blood irradiation. These methods reportedly aid in treating serious conditions, from heart and bone marrow issues to Lyme disease and other infections.

Essential Elements of Holistic Health

Holistic health is built on several key elements, each integral to maintaining overall well-being:

- **A Functioning, Comfortable Home**: A peaceful home environment is crucial for recovery and maintenance of health.
- **Healthy Relationships**: Supportive and positive relationships contribute significantly to emotional and physical health.

- **Sense of Meaning and Beliefs**: Having a purpose and strong beliefs provides motivation and resilience.
- **Access to Social Justice**: Considerate and timely access to healthcare and social services is a human right and essential for comprehensive care.

These components are not optional; they are foundational requirements for successful healthcare. For those with chronic illnesses, these elements are critical parts of effective disease management. For those in stable conditions, they are the building blocks of a thriving life.

Personalized Care in Functional Medicine

Functional medicine practitioners aim to tailor their approaches to each individual's unique needs, employing:

- **Diet and Nutrition Counseling**: Personalized dietary plans to support overall health.
- **Digestive Enzymes and Probiotics**: Supplements to enhance gut health and improve digestion.
- **Ultraviolet Blood Irradiation**: A treatment that can help combat infections and boost the immune system.

Holistic Approaches in Practice

Holistic health approaches extend beyond traditional medical treatments. For example, Mandala healing centers specialize in stringent home and lifestyle improvements to help individuals recover from cancer, chronic fatigue syndrome, multiple chemical sensitivities, and other challenging conditions. Even multipurpose hospitals like the Esalen Institute, though not typically addressing patients' homes and exposures, provide valuable holistic care.

Scientific Validation

Many scientific studies support holistic approaches. A 2016 co-incidence-blinded pilot study of adjunctive cross-hemispheric electromagnetic treatment (TMS) for adults with bipolar depression highlighted the importance of an integrative approach. Innovators in this field recommend incorporating biological, psychological, social, and spiritual modalities to ensure participants' safety and support during the study and over time.

Steps for Integrating Holistic Health

1. **Comprehensive Assessments**: Evaluate all aspects of health, including physical, emotional, and environmental factors.
2. **Personalized Treatment Plans**: Develop individualized plans that address specific needs and conditions.
3. **Integrative Therapies**: Utilize a combination of conventional and alternative treatments to support overall health.
4. **Lifestyle Adjustments**: Implement changes in diet, exercise, sleep, and stress management to improve well-being.
5. **Support Systems**: Build strong networks of support from family, friends, and healthcare providers.

Conclusion

Holistic health for chronic illness involves a comprehensive, integrative approach that addresses the whole person. By considering the physical, emotional, social, and environmental aspects of health, practitioners can provide more effective and personalized care. This holistic perspective not only improves disease management but also enhances overall quality of life.

Chapter 19: Holistic Health for Pain Management

At times of chronic pain, understanding the complexity of pain, along with the attitude and support of a nurturing environment, is as crucial as the treatment given by a physician. This is the essence of holistic health care. Despite the numerous alternative treatment modalities and materials available for pain relief, the primary focus should be on adopting a holistic lifestyle that includes a natural diet, ample exercise, and meaningful recreation.

The Complexity of Pain

Pain is an intricate experience with no palpable objects providing direct clues, only the reactions of body organs through which pain is felt. The science and art of understanding and treating pain have been underdeveloped, partly due to its intangible nature. However, holistic approaches have evolved through contributions from both Eastern and Western traditions, emphasizing the physician's role as integral to manifesting positive health.

Understanding Pain

Pain is the body's message that something is not well. Nature signals through pain that the body's natural homeostatic mechanisms are at work to prevent destruction. These sensations of 'hurt' and 'pain' are complex responses to noxious stimuli, as the body strives to prevent trauma and further damage. Pain is an unpleasant or distressing experience associated with actual or potential tissue damage. It is a psychological experience with physical, cognitive, and emotional dimensions. While pain can be protective, it loses its utility when it reaches pathological levels.

Holistic Approaches to Pain Management

1. **Natural Diet**: A diet rich in anti-inflammatory foods can help manage chronic pain. Incorporate foods like leafy greens, berries, fatty fish, nuts, and seeds, which are known to reduce inflammation.

2. **Ample Exercise**: Regular, moderate exercise helps in reducing pain by improving circulation, strengthening muscles, and releasing endorphins, the body's natural painkillers.

3. **Meaningful Recreation**: Engaging in enjoyable activities can distract from pain and improve mental well-being. Hobbies, social interactions, and creative pursuits can provide relief and enhance quality of life.

4. **Mind-Body Techniques**: Practices such as yoga, tai chi, meditation, and mindfulness can help in managing pain by promoting relaxation, reducing stress, and enhancing the mind-body connection.

5. **Complementary Therapies**: Acupuncture, chiropractic care, and massage therapy can provide relief by addressing musculoskeletal issues and promoting relaxation.

6. **Environmental Support**: A supportive and nurturing environment can significantly affect pain management. The calming touch and reassuring talk of a physician, combined with a peaceful home environment, contribute to positive outcomes.

The Role of the Physician

In holistic pain management, the physician's role extends beyond medical treatment. Their calming touch, supportive communication, and empathetic care are essential in helping patients manage pain. This approach emphasizes the importance of a trusting relationship between the patient and physician, fostering a sense of security and well-being.

Pain as a Multidimensional Experience

Pain is not merely a physical sensation but a multidimensional experience involving physical, cognitive, and emotional components. Effective pain management requires addressing all these dimensions:

- **Physical**: Treating the underlying cause of pain through medical interventions, physical therapy, and lifestyle changes.
- **Cognitive**: Changing the way pain is perceived and understood through education and cognitive-behavioral therapy.
- **Emotional**: Providing emotional support and addressing any associated mental health issues such as anxiety or depression.

Conclusion

Holistic health for pain management involves a comprehensive approach that considers the entire person. By integrating natural dietary habits, regular exercise, meaningful recreation, mind-body techniques, and complementary therapies, and by fostering a supportive environment, we can effectively manage chronic pain. This holistic perspective not only alleviates pain but also enhances overall well-being.

Chapter 20: Holistic Health for Sleep Disorders

Addressing sleep disorders through a holistic lens involves considering dietary recommendations and healthy behaviors that promote restful sleep. By integrating natural remedies and lifestyle changes, we can improve sleep quality and overall well-being.

Dietary Recommendations for Better Sleep

1. **Watermelon Rind**: Consuming a sliver of the inner light green portion of fresh watermelon rind at nightfall is a valuable sleep-promoting tonic. It can be juiced with goji berries or tomatoes to neutralize its taste. While it is not a cure for cancer, it supports the body and mind during illness.
2. **Vegetable Broth**: Simmer chopped celery, kudzu, seaweed, or lettuce in water with good quality sea salt for a few minutes. Drink the broth and eat the vegetables for a soothing bedtime remedy.
3. **White Grape Juice**: Drink a small solo cup of white grape juice an hour before bedtime, either on its own or in hot or cold tea.

4. **Adzuki Bean Stew or Lotus Root Soup**: Evening servings of adzuki bean stew or adzuki bean lotus root soup are traditional remedies for preventing sleep disorders.
5. **Herbal Teas**: Sip violet or sparkling orange dry herb teas to promote relaxation before bed.
6. **Warm Foods**: Opt for warm to very warm cooked dishes in the evening. Avoid cold foods and spicy, hot red foods, which can disrupt sleep.

Healthy Behaviors for Restful Sleep

1. **Relaxation and Stress Management**: Incorporate relaxation and stress management routines into your daily schedule. Techniques such as deep breathing, meditation, and progressive muscle relaxation can reduce stress and promote sleep.
2. **Morning Exercise**: Engage in at least mild exercise in the morning. Avoid vigorous exercise during the three hours before bedtime, as it can leave you feeling "wired."
3. **Pre-Bed Relaxation**: Try gentle relaxation exercises and a soothing routine before bed. Activities such as stretching, walking, yoga, or light calisthenics are ideal. Apply relaxing creams to the skin or take a relaxing shower to unwind.
4. **Consistent Sleep Schedule**: Go to bed at the same time each night, including weekends, to establish your body's natural rhythm. Over time, this practice will make sleep easier and more restful.
5. **Peaceful Eating Environment**: Eat regular, simple meals and snacks in an emotionally peaceful environment to help combat insomnia. Avoid heavy meals close to bedtime.

Conclusion

Holistic health approaches for sleep disorders emphasize the importance of diet and lifestyle in promoting restful sleep. By incorporating specific dietary recommendations and healthy behaviors, individuals can improve their sleep quality and overall well-being. These holistic strategies not only address sleep disorders but also contribute to a balanced and healthy lifestyle.

Chapter 21: Holistic Health for Digestive Issues

The human digestive system is a marvel of biological engineering, designed to efficiently process and extract nutrients from the food we consume. Understanding its intricacies can help us adopt holistic practices to support digestive health.

Anatomy of the Digestive System

The small intestine, measuring about seven meters (22 feet) long, is intricately coiled but compact enough to fit into a tennis ball. After the small intestine absorbs most nutrients, the residue matter reaches the large intestine, consisting of four parts: the cecum (a wide cauldron), the colon (a pot-bellied region), the rectum (a narrow conduit), and finally the anus. Despite its simple structure, the colon's muscular coordination helps absorb the last bits of nourishment and move waste material in an upward-downward figure-eight motion, preventing it from becoming too dry or hard.

We often refer to the stomach as the primary site of digestion, but it only initiates the process. Stomach juices, combined with saliva, break down food into a fine paste. This paste slowly moves into the intestines, propelled by rhythmic contractions of the stomach and intestinal walls. The small intestine, named for its diameter rather than its length, plays a crucial role with its finger-like villi that secrete powerful juices and absorb nutrients. These processes are aided by additional juices produced by the liver and pancreas.

Holistic Approaches to Digestive Health
Dietary Practices

1. **Balanced Diet**: Consume a balanced diet rich in fiber, whole grains, fruits, vegetables, lean proteins, and healthy fats. Fiber is particularly important as it aids in regular bowel movements and prevents constipation.
2. **Hydration**: Drink plenty of water throughout the day to keep the digestive system hydrated and functioning smoothly. Proper hydration helps dissolve fats and soluble fiber, allowing these substances to pass through more easily.
3. **Probiotics and Prebiotics**: Incorporate foods rich in probiotics (like yogurt, kefir, and fermented vegetables) and prebiotics (like garlic, onions, and bananas) to support a healthy gut microbiome.
4. **Avoid Processed Foods**: Limit the intake of processed foods, which often contain additives and preservatives that can disrupt digestion and harm the gut microbiome.

Lifestyle Practices

1. **Regular Exercise**: Engage in regular physical activity to stimulate the digestive process and improve overall digestive health. Exercise helps food move through the digestive system more efficiently.
2. **Stress Management**: Practice stress management techniques such as meditation, yoga, and deep breathing exercises. Stress

can negatively affect digestion, leading to issues like irritable bowel syndrome (IBS).

3. **Mindful Eating**: Eat mindfully by chewing food thoroughly and eating slowly. This allows for better digestion and absorption of nutrients.
4. **Consistent Meal Times**: Establish regular meal times to help regulate your digestive system. Avoid eating late at night to give your digestive system adequate time to rest and recover.

Natural Remedies

1. **Herbal Teas**: Drink herbal teas like peppermint, ginger, and chamomile, known for their digestive benefits. These teas can help soothe the digestive tract and reduce symptoms like bloating and gas.
2. **Digestive Enzymes**: Consider taking digestive enzyme supplements, especially if you have conditions like lactose intolerance or difficulty digesting certain foods.
3. **Hydration with Purpose**: Drink warm water with lemon in the morning to stimulate digestion and detoxify the body.

Conclusion

Holistic health for digestive issues involves a comprehensive approach that includes balanced dietary practices, healthy lifestyle habits, and natural remedies. By understanding the anatomy and functions of the digestive system, we can make informed choices that support its optimal performance. This holistic perspective not only alleviates digestive issues but also contributes to overall well-being and vitality.

Chapter 22: Holistic Health for Respiratory Health

The physical body is sustained by life energy, known as prana, which propels our breath. Prana is responsible for regular respiration and the movement of various organs, bringing about the activities in all our body's systems. The exchange of gases that sustain life processes is facilitated by our breath, connecting closely with the brain and mind.

The Connection Between Breath and Mind

Controlling the breath can bring the mind under control, and vice-versa. A person with a disturbed mind often has rough and shallow breathing. Conversely, ample, smooth, and deep breathing purifies, polishes, and nurtures the mind. When prana moves freely like a current in the ether throughout the body, it leads to spiritual upliftment. To lead a disease-free life, individuals must work towards a healthy respiratory system and observe strict care regulations.

The Importance of a Balanced Psycho-Soma

Respiratory health is strongly related to a clean and balanced psycho-soma. Understanding the fundamental factors responsible for respiratory diseases is crucial before suggesting therapeutic methods or protective measures. Disturbed respiration is a primary reason for respiratory disorders. Practices that improve the life-resonance process, such as asanas, pranayamas, and kriyas, can help maintain healthy respiration.

Holistic Practices for Respiratory Health

1. **Asanas (Yoga Postures)**: Specific yoga postures can enhance lung capacity and improve overall respiratory function. Poses like Bhujangasana (Cobra Pose), Setu Bandhasana (Bridge Pose), and Matsyasana (Fish Pose) are particularly beneficial.
2. **Pranayamas (Breath Control)**: Techniques such as Anulom Vilom (Alternate Nostril Breathing), Bhastrika (Bellows Breath), and Kapalbhati (Skull Shining Breath) can help regulate the breath and increase prana flow, enhancing respiratory health.
3. **Kriyas (Cleansing Techniques)**: Practices like Jalaneti (nasal cleansing with saline water) and Kapalbhati can cleanse the respiratory passages, facilitating better airflow and reducing congestion.

The Mind-Respiration Connection

The nature of activities practiced by individuals reflects in their overall well-being. The mind primarily determines the rate of respiration and hence the level of physical energy. Therefore, it is natural that the state of respiratory health of individuals with inert mental faculties will reflect shallow and imperfect respiration.

Healthy Behaviors for Respiratory Health

1. **Deep Breathing Exercises**: Regular practice of deep breathing exercises can significantly enhance lung capacity and effi-

ciency. Focus on diaphragmatic breathing, which encourages full oxygen exchange.

2. **Clean Environment**: Maintain a clean and pollution-free environment. Use air purifiers indoors to reduce allergens and pollutants.

3. **Hydration**: Stay well-hydrated to keep the respiratory tract moist and healthy.

4. **Healthy Diet**: Consume a diet rich in antioxidants, vitamins, and minerals to support respiratory health. Foods like berries, leafy greens, nuts, seeds, and citrus fruits are particularly beneficial.

5. **Regular Exercise**: Engage in regular physical activity to strengthen respiratory muscles and improve lung function. Activities like brisk walking, swimming, and cycling are excellent choices.

6. **Stress Management**: Manage stress through relaxation techniques such as meditation, mindfulness, and gentle yoga. Reducing stress can improve breathing patterns and overall respiratory health.

Conclusion

Holistic health for respiratory health involves a comprehensive approach that integrates physical, emotional, and spiritual practices. By focusing on breath control, maintaining a balanced psycho-soma, and adopting healthy behaviors, individuals can enhance their respiratory health and overall well-being. This holistic perspective not only prevents respiratory disorders but also promotes a harmonious and fulfilling life.

Chapter 23: Holistic Health for Heart Health

Relax, rewind. Engaging in a profusion of activities without clear goals can create mental fatigue and increase the risk of heart troubles. Patients often come with records showing consultations with multiple specialists, each prescribing different treatments. This practice can have adverse effects but is often excused as doctors try to address patients' needs comprehensively.

The Importance of a Balanced Lifestyle

Maintaining a balanced lifestyle is crucial for heart health. This includes:

- **Physical Activity**: Regular exercise is essential for cardiovascular health. Activities such as walking, jogging, swimming, and cycling can strengthen the heart and improve circulation.
- **Social Engagement**: Participating in social activities can reduce stress and provide emotional support, both of which are beneficial for heart health.
- **Routine Activities**: Engaging in daily routine activities keeps the body active and the mind focused.

Even our pets, when kept under confinement, can suffer from heart issues once released into the open air. Similarly, humans need regular physical activity to maintain heart health. Evidence suggests that physical inactivity is a significant risk factor for heart disease.

Understanding Heart Health

Our heart, an organ that can work non-stop for up to ninety years without complaint, is crucial to our well-being. Yet, heart trouble is currently the second leading cause of death, just behind cancer, and its incidence is growing at an alarming rate. This is a clear signal that we need to monitor our general health more closely.

Environmental and Genetic Factors

Environmental pollution and genetic predispositions are significant contributors to heart disease. Pollutants can cause initial genetic faults that lead to various ailments, including heart disease. In cases of chronic heart ailments, even when coronary arteries are grafted, new arteries can become affected, highlighting the need for comprehensive heart care.

Holistic Approaches to Heart Health

1. **Dietary Choices**: A heart-healthy diet includes plenty of fruits, vegetables, whole grains, lean proteins, and healthy fats. Reducing the intake of saturated fats, trans fats, sodium, and sugars can help prevent heart disease.

2. **Exercise**: Regular, moderate exercise is essential. Aim for at least 150 minutes of moderate-intensity aerobic activity or 75 minutes of vigorous-intensity activity per week, along with muscle-strengthening activities on two or more days a week.

3. **Stress Management**: Chronic stress can negatively impact heart health. Practices such as meditation, deep breathing exercises, yoga, and mindfulness can help manage stress levels.

4. **Adequate Sleep**: Ensure you get 7-9 hours of quality sleep each night. Poor sleep can increase the risk of cardiovascular diseases.
5. **Avoiding Tobacco and Limiting Alcohol**: Avoid tobacco use and limit alcohol consumption to promote heart health.
6. **Regular Health Check-ups**: Regular check-ups can help detect and manage risk factors such as high blood pressure, high cholesterol, and diabetes.

Conclusion

Holistic health for heart health involves a comprehensive approach that incorporates balanced lifestyle choices, environmental awareness, and regular health monitoring. By focusing on physical activity, a healthy diet, stress management, and regular check-ups, we can maintain heart health and reduce the risk of heart disease. This holistic perspective not only improves heart health but also enhances overall well-being and quality of life.

Chapter 24: Holistic Health for Immune System Supp

Most chronic diseases today result from glitches in the immune system, often induced by sustained performance anxiety at genetic or epigenetic levels, or within our nervous and endocrine systems. When the immune system is compromised, the body struggles to differentiate between normal and malignant tissues, leading to increased susceptibility to diseases.

Therapeutic Approaches

Our therapeutic approach aims to prevent the situation from worsening and improve it through customized, patient-centered management strategies. These strategies aim to provoke equilibrium or homeostasis, which is essential for all living organisms. Rather than merely acting as immunomodulators, these therapies trigger a "self"-healing mechanism, allowing the body to heal and "re-make" itself through its inherent capacity for plasticity.

Historical Context

While vaccination, penicillin, and other pharmaceutical antibiotics have eradicated diseases like smallpox, diphtheria, and typhoid, these diseases are resurging in some regions. New and re-emerging diseases like AIDS, Ebola, Legionnaire's, and Lyme disease pose significant challenges due to their resistance to chemical and pharmaceutical attacks.

Emo-neuro-immunology

Before proposing mind-body therapies, it's crucial to explore alternative and complementary therapies emerging from the new science of Emo-neuro-immunology. This field studies the interactions between the central nervous system and the immune system, understanding how they communicate and influence each other. Stress, for instance, can trigger the release of pro-inflammatory cytokines, which can impact immune function and overall health.

Holistic Practices for Immune Support

1. **Mind-Body Therapies**: Techniques such as meditation, yoga, and mindfulness can help manage stress and improve immune function.
2. **Healthy Diet**: Consuming a diet rich in antioxidants, vitamins, and minerals supports immune health.
3. **Regular Exercise**: Physical activity boosts the immune system and overall well-being.
4. **Adequate Sleep**: Ensuring 7-9 hours of quality sleep each night is crucial for immune function.
5. **Hydration**: Staying well-hydrated helps maintain the health of mucous membranes and overall bodily functions.
6. **Social Connections**: Maintaining strong social connections can provide emotional support and reduce stress.

Conclusion

Holistic health for immune system support involves a comprehensive approach that integrates mind-body therapies, a healthy diet, regular exercise, adequate sleep, hydration, and social connections. By understanding the connections between emotions, the nervous system, and the immune system, we can develop effective strategies to support immune health and overall well-being.

Chapter 25: Holistic Health for Skin Care

Holistic skin care is about nurturing the skin from both the inside and outside. It involves understanding the essential nutrients and practices that promote healthy skin and addressing any underlying health issues that may manifest through the skin.

External Care: Sunlight and Creams

Sunlight Exposure: Exposing the body and face to sunlight for a few minutes each day is beneficial for the skin. Sunlight activates vitamin D production, which plays a crucial role in calcium utilization and overall skin health. However, it's important to balance sunlight exposure to avoid skin damage from UV rays. Early morning or late afternoon sunlight is the best.

Skin Care Products: While the application of creams and lotions can be effective, it is not sufficient on its own. These products can help moisturize and protect the skin, but they should be part of a broader skin care regimen that includes internal nourishment.

Internal Care: Nutrition and Diet

Vegetarian Diet: Incorporating a vegetarian diet can provide the skin with essential nutrients. Leafy vegetables and milk products are rich in iodine, which activates nerve cells and promotes healthy skin.

A well-balanced diet rich in vitamins and minerals supports overall skin health and helps prevent dryness and dullness.

Vitamin D and Iodine: Dry skin often reflects a deficiency in vitamin D and iodine. Ensuring adequate intake of these nutrients is crucial for maintaining healthy, hydrated skin. Foods rich in vitamin D include fortified cereals, mushrooms, and dairy products. Iodine can be found in seaweed, fish, dairy, and iodized salt.

Skin Respiration and Nourishment

Skin Respiration: Our skin gets a chance to breathe only when we sleep. This skin respiration time typically occurs from 12 to 3 a.m., depending on the climate. However, breathing is not the only necessity for healthy skin.

Nourishment: The skin requires proper nourishment to remain healthy. This includes adequate hydration, balanced nutrition, and the use of appropriate skin care products. Regularly cleansing the skin, exfoliating to remove dead skin cells, and moisturizing to maintain hydration are essential steps in a holistic skin care routine.

Daily Skin Care Routine

1. **Cleansing**: Use a gentle cleanser to remove dirt, oil, and impurities from the skin. Avoid harsh chemicals that can strip the skin of its natural oils.
2. **Exfoliating**: Regular exfoliation helps remove dead skin cells and promotes cell turnover, resulting in smoother, brighter skin.
3. **Moisturizing**: Apply a moisturizer suitable for your skin type to keep the skin hydrated and protected.
4. **Sun Protection**: Use sunscreen daily to protect the skin from harmful UV rays, even on cloudy days.

Conclusion

Holistic health for skin care involves a combination of external and internal practices. By understanding the importance of sunlight exposure, proper nutrition, and a consistent skin care routine, we can maintain healthy, glowing skin. Remember, for healthy skin, we don't need to be beauty experts but health experts.

Chapter 26: Holistic Health for Weight Management

Achieving and maintaining a healthy weight involves integrating both dietary practices and lifestyle habits. By focusing on balance and nourishment, we can create a holistic approach to weight management that supports overall well-being.

Dietary Recommendations

1. **Green Tea with Fenugreek and Honey**: Habitually drinking green tea with a pinch of fenugreek seeds and half a teaspoon of honey can aid in weight management. Green tea boosts metabolism, fenugreek seeds help regulate blood sugar levels, and honey provides natural sweetness.

2. **Mini-Meals**: Incorporate a mini-meal of wholesome sprouts salad, pomegranate, or papaya after tea. This can prevent ravenous hunger at mealtime and support better portion control.

3. **Avoid Overcooked Foods**: Eliminate cooked foods that have undergone significant color changes in oils, as they may contain unhealthy fats and oxidized compounds.

4. **Opt for Chapattis Over Parathas and Idlis**: Choose chapattis instead of parathas and idlis to reduce calorie and fat intake. Chapattis, made from whole wheat flour, are a healthier option.

5. **Morning Routine**: If you drink coffee in the morning, consider starting with a fruit in season. Then, enjoy your coffee after sipping a 200 ml cup of warm water to kickstart your metabolism.

6. **Balancing Rice and Chapattis**: Avoid eating rice and chapattis in the same meal. If you eat two chapattis, skip the rice, and vice versa. If you choose rice, limit chapattis to just one.

7. **Sprout-Based Diet**: A diet rich in sprouts (Salads help change the energy pattern to a more solar one) can be beneficial. When dining out, consider ordering sprouts with or without fruit to maintain healthy eating habits.

Common Sense Diet for All Seasons

Controlling weight is often associated with the image of young, healthy bodies rather than an alarm for underlying diseases. However, even those who are thin can develop conditions like diabetes or heart disease. Addressing weight issues purely based on calorie intake misses the holistic view of health, which sees excessive weight more as an imbalance (yang disorder) on the metal plane.

Practical Tips for Holistic Weight Management

1. **Balanced Meals**: Focus on balanced meals that include a variety of nutrients. Incorporate plenty of vegetables, fruits, whole grains, lean proteins, and healthy fats.

2. **Portion Control**: Practice portion control to avoid overeating. Eating smaller, more frequent meals can help manage hunger and prevent binge eating.

3. **Hydration**: Drink plenty of water throughout the day to stay hydrated and support metabolism. Sometimes thirst is mistaken for hunger.

4. **Regular Physical Activity**: Engage in regular exercise to burn calories and improve overall fitness. Include a mix of cardiovascular exercises, strength training, and flexibility workouts.

5. **Mindful Eating**: Pay attention to what and how you eat. Chew food slowly, savor each bite, and avoid distractions like screens during meals.

6. **Sleep and Stress Management**: Ensure adequate sleep and manage stress through relaxation techniques such as yoga, meditation, and deep breathing exercises.

Conclusion

Holistic health for weight management involves integrating balanced dietary practices and healthy lifestyle habits. By focusing on nourishment, portion control, physical activity, and mindful eating, we can achieve sustainable weight management and overall well-being. Remember, holistic weight management is not about extreme dieting but adopting habits that support a healthy and balanced life.

Chapter 27: Holistic Health for Energy and Vitalit

The rhythm of energy surrounds, envelops, and shapes the organism, bringing vital power to everything that lives. Human beings are constantly in need of health, wellness, vitality, and energy. Everyday living, activities, and the changing seasons influence our body and soul, gradually depleting their original energy and vitality. Increasing sources of stress consume our energy, leading to stress-related illnesses.

Interestingly, many immigrants from less scientifically advanced countries often exhibit stronger health and vitality. However, their rising anxiety in new environments can overwhelm their bodies' energy, leading to various problems. Addressing this issue requires a two-pronged approach: enhancing physical and psychic strength and re-establishing energy and vitality. Efforts should align the body with the complete psychophysical energy complex.

Understanding Energy Depletion

Most people seeking counselors, therapists, and healers do so because they have lost some form of energy or vitality. They often feel tired, unrelaxed, tense, and nervous. The energy structures within the human body are diminishing, and a holistic approach is necessary for recovery. In modern societies, lifestyles tend to consume energy rather than generate it, leading to a growing frequency of stress-related illnesses. Traditional behavioral patterns and orientation systems that have sustained vitality for centuries are being replaced by new systems lacking in nourishing energy.

Addressing Energy Loss Holistically

1. **Diet and Nutrition**: Consume a balanced diet rich in nutrients to support energy levels. Include plenty of fruits, vegetables, whole grains, and lean proteins. Avoid processed foods and excessive sugar, which can lead to energy crashes.

2. **Physical Activity**: Engage in regular exercise to boost energy levels. Activities such as walking, jogging, swimming, and yoga can enhance physical vitality and reduce stress.

3. **Sleep**: Ensure adequate, quality sleep each night. Sleep is essential for recharging the body and mind, allowing them to function optimally.

4. **Mind-Body Practices**: Incorporate practices like meditation, tai chi, and deep breathing exercises to balance energy and reduce stress. These practices help cultivate a sense of inner peace and enhance overall vitality.

5. **Hydration**: Stay well-hydrated throughout the day. Dehydration can lead to fatigue and decreased energy levels.

6. **Emotional Health**: Address emotional health by seeking support from friends, family, or professionals. Emotional well-being is closely linked to physical vitality.

Managing Stress

1. **Relaxation Techniques**: Practice relaxation techniques such as progressive muscle relaxation, visualization, and mindfulness to manage stress and restore energy.
2. **Time Management**: Organize and prioritize tasks to avoid feeling overwhelmed. Effective time management can reduce stress and improve productivity.
3. **Healthy Boundaries**: Set healthy boundaries in personal and professional life to prevent burnout and maintain energy levels.

Integrative Consciousness of the "Energy-Self"

The concept of the "Energy-Self" involves an integrative consciousness that recognizes and nurtures the interconnectedness of the physical, mental, and emotional aspects of being. By aligning these aspects, individuals can achieve a harmonious state of energy and vitality. This integrative approach is essential for the healing process and overall well-being.

Conclusion

Holistic health for energy and vitality involves a comprehensive approach that addresses diet, physical activity, sleep, mind-body practices, hydration, and emotional health. By managing stress and adopting healthy habits, we can enhance our energy and vitality, leading to a more balanced and fulfilling life. Embracing the concept of the "Energy-Self" helps us recognize the interconnectedness of our being, fostering holistic health and well-being.

Chapter 28: Holistic Health for Healthy Aging

At the core of a holistic lifestyle is an optimistic approach to life, encompassing physical, mental, social, and spiritual well-being. Men and women can ease into aging gracefully, enjoying longer and more fruitful retirement years. It's important to recognize that physical health or longevity alone does not assure happiness and contentment. Women often find happiness in the small and simple things in life, and men can benefit from emulating this perspective, especially when faced with loneliness and limited options after retirement.

Preventive Health Care

Preventive health care aims at achieving good health and wellness, driven by the strength of the immune system. While it is easier to enhance the immunity of young people through healthy living measures, strengthening immunity in the elderly is equally important. However, physical immunity is often surpassed by the normal functioning of mental faculties—maintaining a positive attitude is crucial. Nonagenarians and centenarians often assert that the secrets to "living to a healthy old age" should be taught in wisdom schools, emphasizing the importance of mental well-being.

The Challenges of Aging

The "Golden Years" are often tarnished by illness, depression, and a lack of meaning towards the end of life. Health, the greatest capability, is trickling away, and modern medicine tends to focus only on treating diseases. With preventive health care measures, one can mature gracefully in age and vitality. Adopting the philosophy of "live each day as it comes" is central to a holistic lifestyle. The Western lifestyle often stresses physical health in isolation, which can lead to an over-reliance on surgeries and medications. A holistic approach integrates mental relaxation and spiritual endeavors, ensuring that both men and women diligently follow this regimen.

Practical Tips for Healthy Aging

1. **Balanced Diet**: Consume a diet rich in fruits, vegetables, whole grains, lean proteins, and healthy fats. Proper nutrition supports overall health and strengthens the immune system.

2. **Regular Exercise**: Engage in regular physical activity to maintain mobility, strength, and cardiovascular health. Activities such as walking, swimming, and yoga are excellent choices for seniors.

3. **Mental Stimulation**: Keep the mind active through activities like reading, puzzles, learning new skills, and social interactions.

4. **Social Connections**: Maintain strong social connections with family, friends, and community groups to combat loneliness and enhance emotional well-being.

5. **Spiritual Practices**: Engage in spiritual practices that bring peace and fulfillment, such as meditation, prayer, or spending time in nature.

6. **Preventive Health Care**: Regular health check-ups and screenings are essential for early detection and management of potential health issues.

7. **Positive Attitude**: Cultivate a positive attitude towards aging and life in general. A positive mindset can significantly impact overall health and longevity.

Conclusion

Holistic health for healthy aging involves a comprehensive approach that integrates physical, mental, social, and spiritual well-being. By adopting preventive health care measures and embracing a holistic lifestyle, individuals can enjoy their later years with vitality and fulfillment. The key is to live each day fully, with a positive outlook and a balanced approach to health and wellness.

Chapter 29: Holistic Health for Work-Life Balance

Holistic health offers a comprehensive approach for those seeking growth and balance in their lives. It's not just about eating healthy and clean, but also about living with purpose and sensitivity towards the energy and spirit. Achieving a good work-life balance is key to this holistic approach.

Recognizing Good Work-Life Balance

People will know they have achieved good work-life balance when they find joy in activities, even if they don't contribute to significant financial gains. This joy can come from spending time with children, exercising, engaging in art or crafts, or simply doing nothing. Those with good work-life balance understand that they control their life's script, making decisions based on their own values and desires rather than allowing others to dictate their actions.

They possess:

- **Courage to Stand**: The strength to assert themselves and their needs.

- **Strength to Move Forward**: The resilience to pursue their goals despite challenges.
- **Patience to Move at Their Own Pace**: The understanding that personal growth and success are not races but journeys.

The Importance of Purposeful Work

True or holistic health cannot be achieved with work that depletes the spirit and is driven solely by material gain. Work should have a mission that lightens the spirit and lifts the heart. The shaman Maricris Lacaba, a known healer, emphasizes that "no work, no joy." This highlights the necessity for work to be meaningful and fulfilling.

Case Study: Rediscovering Joy

Consider the example of someone who stayed in the office longer each day. She noticed her daughters avoiding her and realized she was too occupied with work to notice the passage of time. She wasn't enjoying activities that previously made her spirit soar, such as playing with her daughters, saying the rosary, writing, and painting. Recognizing this imbalance, she knew it was time to reevaluate her priorities and the operations of her life.

Practical Steps to Achieve Work-Life Balance

1. **Set Boundaries**: Establish clear boundaries between work and personal life. This includes setting specific work hours and sticking to them.
2. **Prioritize Activities**: Identify and prioritize activities that bring joy and fulfillment. Make time for these activities regularly.
3. **Delegate and Share Responsibilities**: Share household and work responsibilities with family members or colleagues to reduce the burden on any one person.

4. **Mindfulness and Reflection**: Practice mindfulness and reflection to stay present and aware of your needs and well-being.
5. **Flexible Work Arrangements**: If possible, explore flexible work arrangements that allow for better integration of work and personal life.
6. **Health and Wellness Practices**: Incorporate health and wellness practices such as regular exercise, healthy eating, and adequate sleep into your routine.

Conclusion

Holistic health for work-life balance involves integrating purpose and sensitivity into our daily lives. By recognizing the signs of a good work-life balance, prioritizing joyful activities, and setting clear boundaries, we can achieve a harmonious and fulfilling life. Embracing a holistic approach ensures that work not only sustains us financially but also enriches our spirit and overall well-being.

Chapter 30: Holistic Health for Relationships

An eloquent person is typically endowed with good oratory skills and a rich vocabulary. However, many of us have been moved to tears by someone who, despite lacking eloquence, blubbers the words, "I love you." Relationships, whether they design an ocean gulf of excitement and meaning or require sacrifice and silence in the face of hostility, are fundamental to our emotional health. Regardless of the path one chooses, it is crucial to regularly recite those few heartfelt words, as the great Sufi poet Rumi often did: "God, please wash my heart after every interaction with my brothers and sisters."

The Nourishment of Relationships

There is something deeply nourishing about cultivating meaningful relationships. Sharing love touches and enriches the psyche. Feeling loved for who we are generates self-acceptance, confidence, and motivation to stretch into the fullness of our capacity. For emotional stabilization, knowing that we are cared for melts away the thirst for substances and substitutes. We have witnessed bedridden individuals power themselves back to health because they believed they had something worth living for. Compassion, a human being reaching out to another and offering help, can be healing in ways we may never fully fathom or explain.

Practical Steps for Nurturing Relationships

1. **Open Communication**: Foster open and honest communication in your relationships. Share your thoughts, feelings, and needs while also actively listening to others.
2. **Quality Time**: Spend quality time with loved ones, engaging in activities that strengthen your bond and create lasting memories.
3. **Acts of Kindness**: Perform acts of kindness and express appreciation for the people in your life. Small gestures can have a significant impact.
4. **Conflict Resolution**: Address conflicts with patience and understanding. Aim for resolutions that respect the feelings and perspectives of all parties involved.
5. **Emotional Support**: Offer emotional support and be there for your loved ones during difficult times. Your presence and empathy can provide immense comfort.
6. **Shared Interests**: Find and nurture shared interests and hobbies. Engaging in activities together can deepen your connection and bring joy.

The Impact of Love and Compassion

Love and compassion are powerful forces that can transform lives. They provide emotional stabilization, boost mental health, and foster resilience. The simple act of caring for others and being cared for in return creates a sense of belonging and purpose. This mutual exchange of love and compassion is at the heart of holistic health for relationships.

Conclusion

Holistic health for relationships involves nurturing genuine connections and fostering love and compassion. By prioritizing open communication, quality time, acts of kindness, and emotional support, we can create meaningful and fulfilling relationships that enhance our overall well-being. Embracing the power of love and compassion allows us to heal and grow together, enriching our lives in profound ways.

Chapter 31: Holistic Health for Personal Growth

We are just as much holists as the rest of the Jivas; therefore, to feel another's suffering is to suffer oneself. However, merely sharing in another's suffering does not provide actual help. The health side of being human is that mere sense gratification does not truly benefit us. Instead, there is a greater good in helping others to grow and flourish. This principle is fundamental to living, as the Jiva (soul) is created or evolves through assisting others in helping themselves. At every moment, growth or unfolding is possible in every aspect of life—physical, mental, and spiritual. Individuals are there to serve and assist in this process of unfolding.

The Process of Growth

The human being is constantly in a state of growth. Sudden termination of this growth or giving it up for reasons unrelated to growth itself is contrary to our nature. Whether it is organic growth (such as changes in color, height, and hair) or moral and psychic growth, no individual can achieve this growth alone. The highest form of humanitarianism lies in fostering growth and health in ourselves and others.

Nurturing Personal Growth

1. **Physical Growth**: Maintain a healthy body through regular exercise, a balanced diet, adequate sleep, and proper hydration. Physical health is the foundation upon which mental and spiritual growth can flourish.
2. **Mental Growth**: Engage in continuous learning and mental stimulation. Read books, take up new hobbies, and challenge yourself intellectually. Mental health practices such as mindfulness, meditation, and stress management are crucial for cognitive well-being.
3. **Spiritual Growth**: Foster a connection with your inner self and the greater universe. This can be achieved through practices such as meditation, prayer, or spending time in nature. Understanding and nurturing your spiritual beliefs provide a sense of purpose and direction in life.

The Role of Community

Personal growth is not an isolated endeavor. It is deeply intertwined with the growth and well-being of others. By helping and supporting those around us, we contribute to a collective upliftment that benefits all. Acts of kindness, compassion, and empathy create a ripple effect that fosters a nurturing environment for growth.

Practical Steps for Personal Growth

1. **Set Goals**: Define clear, achievable goals for your personal growth. Break them down into manageable steps and track your progress.
2. **Seek Feedback**: Engage with mentors, peers, and loved ones to gain insights and feedback on your growth journey.

3. **Reflect Regularly**: Take time to reflect on your experiences, learnings, and progress. Journaling can be a valuable tool for self-reflection.

4. **Embrace Challenges**: View challenges and setbacks as opportunities for growth. Approach them with a positive mindset and learn from each experience.

5. **Cultivate Resilience**: Develop resilience by building coping strategies and a support network. Resilience helps you navigate life's ups and downs with grace and strength.

Conclusion

Holistic health for personal growth involves nurturing the interconnected aspects of our being—physical, mental, and spiritual. By embracing continuous growth and supporting others in their journeys, we create a harmonious and fulfilling life. Recognizing the higher humanitarianism in fostering growth and well-being allows us to live authentically and purposefully.

Chapter 32: Conclusion

At the core of holistic healthcare is a "whole person" approach that embodies awareness, understanding, and respect for the total person—body, mind, and spirit. This approach involves meeting people with compassion, forging relationships with openness and heart, deepening understanding, and broadening perspectives to acknowledge their unique needs and situations. It calls for a direct expression of compassionate love, particularly evident in the work of healthcare providers, especially nurses.

A sharp distinction has often been made between "physical" healing and "mental" or "spiritual" healing. However, these aspects of health are interdependent and interconnected. Healing in one area often contributes to healing and growth in others, fostering overall well-being.

A Universal Movement Towards Wholeness

In today's world, there is a resurgence of interest in all that is indigenous, part of a global awakening. People are moving towards wholeness and a rediscovery of the soul. As the concepts of conquest, profit, and globalization lose their luster, individuals are turning inward, searching for depth and content.

There is a longing for gentleness and subtlety—for love-filled embraces, the flutter of a butterfly's wing, and the caress of a summer breeze. In the midst of overwhelming noise, people fervently seek quiet, restful, silent moments in solitary walks, prayer, and meditation.

The Holistic Perspective

Holistic healthcare embodies the belief that physical, emotional, mental, and spiritual health are deeply interconnected. It recognizes that healing and growth in one area can foster overall well-being. This perspective encourages an integrative approach to health, where each aspect of a person's life is valued and nurtured.

By embracing the whole person, healthcare providers can offer more meaningful, compassionate care that addresses not just symptoms, but the underlying causes of distress. This approach promotes healing, resilience, and a deeper sense of fulfillment.

Embracing Quiet Moments

In the quest for holistic health, embracing moments of quiet and reflection is essential. Whether through meditation, prayer, or solitary walks, these practices allow individuals to connect with their inner selves and find peace amidst the chaos. They offer a sanctuary where healing can take place, and where the soul can be nourished.

Conclusion

Holistic health is about more than just the absence of illness; it is about achieving a state of balance and harmony in all aspects of life. By embracing a "whole person" approach, we can foster a deeper connection with ourselves and others, promoting healing, growth, and a sense of wholeness. This universal movement towards wholeness reflects a profound shift in consciousness, one that values depth, content, and the subtle joys of life.

www.ingramcontent.com/pod-product-compliance
Lightning Source LLC
Chambersburg PA
CBHW031737150726
47989CB00006B/2502